ICD-10 Code Breaking: Understanding ICD-10

A Last Minute Guide to ICD-10 for Coders, Non-Coders, and Clinical Teams

Christopher Draven

ISBN: 1517446562
ISBN-13: 978-1517446567

PUBLISHER'S NOTE

This book was released as a last minute guide to the United States implementation of ICD-10. The content is based on information that was available previous to the ICD-10 implementation and should not be used as a guide on how to assign medical diagnosis codes.

INTRODUCTION

ICD-10 is coming…and you couldn't feel more like Jon Snow ("You know nothing, Jon Snow…"). Your head is spinning with news coverage and various emails from training vendors heralding a world where insurance companies are going to deny every claim and the whole healthcare system will shut down!

Any change comes with bumps and bruises, but as you will learn in the following pages, ICD-10 is not an insurmountable enemy.

The purpose of this book is to help fill those gaps, give out clear and correct information, and set you on the path to discerning between fact and fiction.

ICD-10 has been called the "biggest change in modern health care since the implementation of HIPAA."

WHAT YOU CAN EXPECT

A quick search of Amazon.com shows that there are plenty of ICD-10 resources available out there. So, why would you want to spend a few bucks on this book?

The cost of many ICD-10 resources on Amazon.com are $50.00 or more. Resources that are in the $10.00 or lower price range are typically extremely specialized (focusing on codes for one medical specialty).

This resource is a generalist's book. Take a moment to review the table of contents. You will see that a variety of ICD-10 related subjects are covered. Each chapter provides an appropriate level of detail so you fully understand the topic.

At the end of this book you will be able to:
-   Understand the logic of how ICD-10 codes are structured
-   Recognize an ICD-10 code
-   Identify the areas of biggest challenge in the ICD-10 implementation
-   Determine the difference between Facts and Myths about the ICD-10 code set
-   Help others start preparing for the 2015 ICD-10 transition

WHAT THIS BOOK IS NOT

This book may not be for you if you are:
-   a certified coder who has prepared for ICD-10
-   a popular ICD-10 blogger
-   someone who has worked on a project to implement ICD-10 changes for your employer

This book is meant to help with general information regarding the new code set, answer some frequent questions, and look at some of the biggest impacts.

Important Note: By reading this book you will not be able to proficiently code in ICD-10.

WHAT ELSE?

For some, a general overview of the ICD-10 code set will not provide enough value. After all, much of the information found within this book is something you could dig through blogs and websites to find. ICD-10 is not a proprietary system of coding owned by a corporation. It is "held in the public trust" as a cross-cultural standard of medical coding.

The code set, and most importantly the truth about the code set, are all in the public domain.

This book is a basic primer for someone who may not know the differences between the truth, and the noise of sensationalist blog posters and news casters. Yes, there are a lot of codes. However, if every other industrialized nation in the world has moved to ICD-10...the United States of America should be able to manage the transition.

This book is presented as a tool to help minimize the amount of research you will need to accomplish to fully understand what is coming.
When you read this book, you will gain a good understanding of the key elements of ICD-10. You will be able to take the knowledge presented here and determine how it will impact your business or processes.

ICD-10 is coming...but you don't need to be caught unaware. After all, it's unlikely your name is Jon Snow.

MEDICAL CODING REVIEW

To start, it is important to understand what is meant by ICD-10.
In training sessions, blogs, and conversations with medical professionals, you will often encounter a blurred line between diagnosis codes and procedure codes.

Diagnosis codes are the codes assigned to specific diseases, disorders, and conditions. Examples could include: Broken arm, Depression, or Animal bite.

Procedure codes are the codes assigned to medical procedures done to heal or cure a diagnosis. Examples could include: Putting a dressing on a wound, prescription medication, or taking an x-ray.

International Classifications of Diseases (ICD)

The International Classifications of Diseases is a coding system that is maintained by the World Health Organization.

News casters will often incorrectly state that the ICD-10 code set is an invention of Medicare. That is simply incorrect. The ICD has been around for several decades (more information on the ICD in the ICD-10 overview).

Healthcare Common Procedure Coding System (HCPCS)

To continue complicating the medical coding landscape, the HCPCS is developed for use in the United States of America and is broken down into various "levels" of code sets. The HCPCS, unlike the ICD, was developed for and by the United States of America.

The HCPCS is maintained by the American Medical Association (AMA) and the Centers for Medicare/Medicaid Services (CMS). The coding system is updated often, with codes for one procedure changing mid-year in some cases – even though the procedure hasn't changed, just the code that is used.

Most professional billers and coders refer to the HCPCS as CPT codes. CPT stands for Current Procedural Terminology. In the "industry" this helps coders easily refer to the different types of codes found within the HCPCS.

Technically, all of the procedure codes in the HCPCS are HCPCS...which to an outsider seems like an obvious statement. Below is a breakdown of the two most common HCPCS levels. Understanding these levels, and how the levels are referred to in the industry, may help you understand why the terminology can get fuzzy.

Level 1: Current Procedural Terminology (CPT)

This level is the largest body of codes within the HCPCS. That is likely the reason most people refer to the HCPCS codes as CPT codes.

CPT codes are the common procedures a physician would use to diagnosis or treat a diagnosis. CPT codes are numeric only. And while there are three categories within the CPT code structure, the most commonly referred to codes are found within the first category. Those codes are broken out into ranges of like procedures. There are six sections of the first CPT code category.

-   **Evaluation and Management**: 99201–99499
-   **Anesthesia**: 00100–01999; 99100–99150
-   **Surgery**: 10000–69990
-   **Radiology**: 70000-79999
-   **Pathology and Laboratory**: 80000–89398
-   **Medicine**: 90281–99099; 99151–99199; 99500–99607

Level 2: Non-Physician Services (DME, J-Code Drugs, etc)

This level (and the other less commonly used levels in the HCPCS) are referred to as HCPCS. These codes are broken down into categories. Each category is assigned a letter. Each code within each category begins with the letter of that category.

HCPCS are non-physician services. A quick look at the HCPCS categories shows that it includes a wide range of possible procedures. HCPCS are alpha-numeric.

- A-codes: Transportation, Medical & Surgical Supplies, Miscellaneous & Experimental
- B-codes: Enteral and Parenteral Therapy
- C-codes: Temporary Hospital Outpatient Prospective Payment System
- D-codes: Dental Procedures
- E-codes: Durable Medical Equipment
- G-codes: Temporary Procedures & Professional Services
- H-codes: Rehabilitative Services
- J-codes: Drugs Administered Other Than Oral Method, Chemotherapy Drugs
- K-codes: Temporary Codes for Durable Medical Equipment Regional Carriers
- L-codes: Orthotic/Prosthetic Procedures
- M-codes: Medical Services
- P-codes: Pathology and Laboratory
- Q-codes: Temporary Codes
- R-codes: Diagnostic Radiology Services
- S-codes: Private Payer Codes
- T-codes: State Medicaid Agency Codes
- V-codes: Vision/Hearing Services

ICD-10 Impact to Procedural Codes

As mentioned earlier in this book, the ICD-10 code set focuses solely on diagnosis codes. The HCPCS and CPT code sets are unaffected by the ICD-10 implementation.

However, as found in ICD-9, there are a group of codes known as the PCS. These codes will be covered in detail later in the book. Briefly, these codes are hospital inpatient procedural codes, and are not used for outpatient physician settings.

ICD-10 OVERVIEW

The history of the ICD is interesting. While many physicians in history codified and categorized various diseases and conditions, few of these methods were widely known or trained. It wasn't until 1893, when a French physician named Jacques Bertillon, introduced his Bertillon Classification of Causes of Death at gathering of statisticians in Chicago, IL. The classification system was immediately adopted by several countries. Based on the idea of breaking down general ailments to localized or specific regions of the body (known as anatomical references), Bertillon's method became the first truly "internationally" accepted system (previously systems were broken down by country and at times by individual cities).

Eventually the system was widely used, and formal revisions and reviews were put in place to keep the system updated and current. Often, systems of other countries were merged with the existing system, growing the scope of the code set.

Since 1900, the ICD has been revisited and revised every 10 years.

The current system, ICD-10, stands for International Classification of Diseases – 10th Revision. And work on the ICD-11 is already underway.

WHAT IS IT FOR?

Understanding where the ICD came from helps you understand the point of such a classification system. As the system came into use, more and more people were traveling. Moving between countries, especially in Europe, often means a complete change in language. And while the first use of the Bertillon Classification system was to track causes of death for statistical measuring by country, it didn't take long for the medical community to see the value in one shared and common language.

When someone is diagnosed with a broken arm in French, the code used is the same code for broken arm in German. This allows the diagnosis to transcend regional barriers.

Operating from the same code set also allows countries to work together to research causes of death and disease. Classifying everything the same way makes tracking down clusters of diseases easier.

Any time you have heard a statistic about a specific disease being the number one killer among people of a certain demographic, that is the ICD in action.

In the United States of America, the ICD has been incorporated in the claims payment processes of insurance companies. An ICD code is required for any claim submitted for reimbursement (from both private and government insurers). The code set is not used in this way in many other countries. Instead, in many countries, the code set is only used to report causes of death.

ICD-9

The ICD-9 code set was released for widespread use in 1975. There are many health care and medical billing professionals who have never used another system. This familiarity, and the integration of the code set in claim payment processes, has made it especially difficult for the United States to comfortably migrate from the ICD-9 to the newer ICD-10.

Many people within in the United States, including some very well-funded medical community organizations, have resisted the migration from ICD-9 to ICD-10. There are some who think the ICD-10 implementation is a device of CMS, like the current requirements of implementing Electronic Medical Records (EMRs), E-Prescribing, Claim Payment Sequestration for Medicare Claims, and so on.

While CMS has put many mandates out there for health care modernization, the ICD-10 code set has been around for some time, and the entire United States, not just those who interact with CMS, are behind the times.

ICD-9 IS OUT OF DATE

Frankly, ICD-9 has run out of space. So many medical advances have been made since the 1970s that are not easily added into the existing structure of ICD-9. Several new diseases have been identified, way of signifying severity, and the ability to differentiate between etiology of various conditions (gestational diabetes and diabetes caused by an underlying condition like pancreatitis do not have the same etiology or method of treatment).

In an age of instant answers on the internet, using an outdated diagnosis code set is silly. Having more information available is the best way to ensure good patient care. ICD-9 has several limitations that can directly impact patient care.

ICD-9 Limitations include:
— No more room in the code set.
— The ICD-9 code set does not allow for a distinction in laterality. This means if you have a broken arm, there is no code to tell you which arm is broken.
— Limited ability to signify the severity of a condition or disease.
— Limited ability to signify the etiology of a condition or disease.
— A confusing use of all coding where the first digit of a code is always a number, unless the digit is a V or an E for some codes that were tacked on.

ICD-10 addresses all of these common issues with ICD-9.

ICD-10

The ICD-10 code set is not brand new. Work began on the revision of ICD-9 in 1983. In 1990, the ICD-10 code set was made available for international use. The first countries to adopt ICD-10 did so in 1992.

The ICD-10 code set has been in use and active since the early 90s. It is an important and unfortunate fact that the United States is the only industrialized nation in the world that has not fully migrated to ICD-10. Added to that injury to American Pride is the fact that ICD-11 is already in development.

List of Countries and when they implemented ICD-10

Country Name	Adopted ICD-10
Canada	2001
Brazil	1998
South Africa	1996
France	1996
United Kingdom	1995
Russia	1999
China	2002
Australia	1998

As you can see, the United States is way behind in the implementation of ICD-10, when compared to so many other nations.

WHY NOT SKIP TO ICD-11?

Critics of moving to ICD-10 often ask, "If moving is so important, why don't we jump over 10 and go straight to ICD-11?"

There are a lot of reasons to move through the code sets in order. Often industry experts state that the move to ICD-11 would take even longer for the United States to get on board. Various groups have indicated the transition to ICD-11 could take the United States into the 2030s before implementation is complete. That number even looks unreal! A migration from ICD-9 to ICD-11 would be an even more traumatic experience for the medical community and insurance industry in the United States.

ICD-10 was released in 1990. The ICD-10-CM (clinical modifications; covered in the next section) was not published until 1995. That code set, the ICD-10-CM, is a huge part of what the United States uses in its use of diagnosis codes. Remember that the ICD is first used for causes of mortality. The use of the code set for diagnosis codes is a secondary use that not all countries participate in.

Even though the ICD-10-CM code set was released and made available for use in mid the 1990s, it wasn't until 2008 that the Department of Health and Human Services proposed a rule that the United States adopt the ICD-10. Twelve years after the code set used by the United States was released by the World Health Organization, the United States decided to investigate the possibility of transitioning.

ICD-11 will not be published for a few more years. Holding off until that code set is published will only set the United States even further behind.

WHAT DOES CMS/MEDICARE HAVE TO SAY ABOUT ICD-10?

CMS has many pages of content on their website dedicated to the "Journey to ICD-10." The content, while topical, is often general and more of an overview than specific instructions. There are some resources that are helpful for small practices or individual providers, however there are limited medical coding or insurance payer implementation resources.

On the website, CMS states a general overview of the differences between ICD-9 and ICD-10 that is pretty good. Below is the information presented on the CMS website (additional notes have been added to provide more clarity around specific topics):

ICD-9	ICD-10
No Laterality	Laterality (Right or Left – accounts for more than 40% of all new codes)
3-5 Digits	7 possible digits
No placeholder character	Uses an "X" placeholder character to minimize confusion. (not in use in all codes)
14,000 codes	69,000 codes
Limited Severity Parameters	Extensive Severity Parameters
Limited Combination Codes	Extensive use of Combination Codes (to better capture diagnosis complexity)
1 type of Excludes Notes	2 types of Excludes Notes (used by medical coders to understand when certain codes are appropriate to use)

The next section is also adapted from the CMS website. The information is broken down into specific categories of reasons why you should prepare for ICD-10.

WHY PREPARE FOR ICD-10?

Reasons to prepare for ICD-10 can be broken down into four categories:

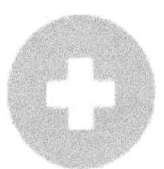

Clinical

- Informs better clinical decisions as better data is documented, collected, and evaluated
- Provides new insights into patients and clinical care due to greater specificity, laterality, and more detailed documentation of patient diseases
- Enables patient segmentation to improve care for higher acuity patients
- Improves tracking of illnesses and severity over time
- Improves public health reporting and helps to track and evaluate the risk of adverse public health events
- Drives greater opportunity for research, trials, and epidemiological studies

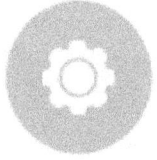

Operational

- Enhances the definition of patient conditions
- Affords more targeted capital investment to meet practice needs Supports practice transition to risk-sharing models with more precise data for patients and populations

Professional

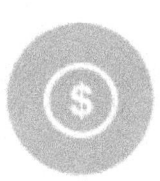

Financial

- Provides clear objective data for credentialing and privileges
- Improves specificity of measures for quality and efficiency reporting
- Aids in the prevention and detection of healthcare fraud and abuse
- Provides more specific data to support physician advocacy of health and public health policy
- Allows better documentation of patient complexity and level of care, supporting reimbursement for care provided
- Provides objective data for peer comparison and utilization benchmarking
- May reduce audit risk exposure by encouraging the use of diagnosis codes with a greater degree of specificity as supported by the clinical documentation

HOW ICD-10 IS STRUCTURED

The ICD-10 code set is a complete departure from the structure of the familiar ICD-9. While the ICD-9 code set was numeric only, the ICD-10 code set is alpha-numeric. This change alone allows for a larger number of possible codes.

Later in the book, you will read how the ICD-10 codes are broken down into component parts. The logic of how the codes are put together is very simple, and will help you in figuring out what various codes mean.

On the surface, the ICD-10 code set is broken into two main components (this is true for those coders and medical professionals who work for organizations within the United States). The two components are ICD-10-CM and ICD-10-PCS.

In addition to the two sets of codes that make up ICD-10, the method to interpreting how to apply codes to a diagnosis has also changed.

In ICD-9, injury codes (called external causes of injury) are grouped by categories of injury or illness. In ICD-10, codes are grouped by the affected body part.

ICD-10-CM

ICD-10-CM is the real star of the show, and will likely be what you are most interested in learning. The CM stands for Clinical Modifications. This category of ICD-10 codes are the diagnostic codes.

The ICD-10-CM is broken down into several sections. Each section contains specific types of diseases that have been grouped together based on etiology or affected system.

The first character in every ICD-10-CM code is represented by a letter. This letter designates which section of the ICD-10-CM code set that code is being pulled from.

For example, you would no longer use 250 to signify all diabetes diagnoses (as it was used in ICD-9). In ICD-10-CM, diabetes can be found in E (for endocrine), O (for obstetrics), and Z (which is not as easy to give a quick mnemonic device to remember, but it is for all other health factors or considerations). This is because diabetes does not have one simple etiology. Diabetes can be a result of endocrine disease (E08-E11), a condition related to a complicated pregnancy (O24), or simply reporting of a personal or family history of diabetes (Z83.3 or Z86.32)

As you can see, understanding the etiology of a disease or condition is key to properly coding in ICD-10. In the past, ICD-9 did not require much in the way of specification around etiology or causation. Simply selecting diabetes unspecified would get your claim paid. However, that mentality is not the best for patient care. When you properly code a patient's illnesses or conditions, other physicians and medical providers are able to key in to the specifics of the patient's diagnosis.

You would not treat gestational diabetes in the same way you would treat type 1 diabetes. However, in ICD-9, you could easily use the same code for both.

ICD-10-CM STRUCTURE

The ICD-10-CM code set is significantly different from the ICD-9 code set. The immediate differences include:

ICD-9	ICD-10
3-5 characters per code	3-7 characters per code
Codes are numeric only (unless using V&E supplemental codes)	Codes are all alphanumeric

The structure to ICD-10 is a very logical progression from left-to-right. This is true for ICD-10-CM and ICD-10-PCS. You will read about ICD-10-PCS in another chapter.

Character	Description
1	This character of an ICD-10-CM code is always a letter. The first digit signifies which of the 21 Chapters the code is taken from. A full list of the ICD-10-CM Chapters can be found later in this book.
2-3	The second and third character before the decimal in an ICD-10-CM code are used to identify the specific condition from within the designated chapter.
Decimal	A decimal point always follows the third character. Together, the first three characters designate the overall diagnosis. Characters 4 through 7 are used to more specifically identify pertinent details about the diagnosis.
4-6	Characters 4 through 6 are used to denote the etiology, site/anatomical location, and manifestation.
7	This character, often called the "7th Character Extension" is used to provide various "extra" information that is vital to fully understanding a diagnosis. The 7th Character Extension is most often used in coding of pregnancy, injury, and poisoning codes, as well as other external causes of morbidity. The character is used to denote: • Episode of Care (initial vs subsequent) • Fracture Type (Open vs Closed; and classification of fracture) • Comma Scale • Trimester • Sequela

Unrelated note about Open and Closed Fractures

As a side note: There are several classification systems that exist for typing fractures. Examples include the Tscherne classification, the Mangled Extremity Severity Scale, AO Fracture scale, and the Hanover scale. ICD-10 has standardized the systems that should be used to classify open and closed fractures.

Open Fractures   Gustilo classification system

Closed Fractures   Salter-Harris classification system

NEW CONCEPTS IN ICD-10

While none of the following concepts are new to health care, they are new additions to the ICD code set requirements. Many of these concepts are required to properly code in ICD-10.

Anatomical Reference
Identifying exactly where in or on the body the injury or infection is located seems like a logical requirement. However, in ICD-9, the exact anatomical reference is not always (or even not often) required.

For the next several terms, we will use the example of a broken arm. In ICD-9, 812.0 is a code used to denote a fractured humerus bone. There are then only three options for anatomical reference: upper end, shaft, and lower end.

In ICD-10, to start there are three possible codes: Upper End S42.2, Shaft S42.3, Lower End S42.4. Once you have determined which section of the humerus bone was broken, then you will need to define the specific anatomical location. A few of the possibilities are listed below:

Lesser tuberosity, greater tuberosity, surgical neck, fracture (avulsion) of lateral epicondyle of humerus, fracture (avulsion) of medial epicondyle of humerus

In addition to these anatomical location possibilities, there are also various break types for each section.

Laterality
As discussed earlier, laterality makes up a large portion of the new codes found within ICD-10. Laterality simply means if something is affecting the left, right, or both sides of the body.

Let's take a broken arm as an example (S42). Which arm is broken, the left (S42.302) or the right (S42.301)? Maybe it is both arms? Laterality is the concept in ICD-10 that will help make clear which arm you are coding.

This coding concept shows up any time an injury or illness may affect both sides of the body (lungs, arms, kidneys, eyes, ears, or any other example of anatomy that is found on both sides of the body).

Instance

Instance is simply whether this is the first time the patient is being seen for this injury, or a subsequent visit. The value in this differentiator is all about patient care.

To continue with the broken arm example, the first visit for treatment of a broken left arm would be the initial encounter (S42.302A). When you visit the physician a few weeks later to check how the break is healing, the physician would submit a subsequent encounter code (S42.302D).

Healing

When considering the Instance concept, you are often required to also consider the Healing concept. This concept is used to signify how the healing of an injury has progressed. This is usually found in the codes for fractures. The concept includes either routine or delayed healing. And to complicate matters further, the healing of an injury is also tied to the way the fracture is healing (in the case of bone fractures). This is designated by either union or nonunion (clinical terms which mean the bone has either reconnected or is still fractured apart). You may also see malunion in the code set (a clinical term that means the bone has reconnected, but in an incorrect manner).

In the example of a broken arm, the S42.302D code has already answered the healing and union/nonunion question. The code signifies the bone is healing appropriately.

Sequela

The term Sequela means that the condition is the consequence of another injury or illness. Meaning, a broken arm caused by a wild pitch in a baseball game is a completely different etiology than a broken arm caused by osteoporosis, or even an automobile accident.

The ability to designate that a condition or injury is directly tied or related to another key diagnosis paints a much clearer picture of the patient's diagnosis. Treating a malunioned broken arm that has healed poorly on a young child who broke their arm playing outside is a much less complicated process than healing the shattered arm bone of an older patient with osteoporosis.

Knowing the causation is all about better patient care.

Etiology

Understanding the cause of an illness, infection, injury, or disease is a vital component to determining how an ailment should be treated. In the other terms listed above, a pattern of etiology seems to crop up every time. This is because patient care is sacrificed when you do not know the cause of a condition.

New Coding Concepts

Beyond the inclusion of clinical concepts into the ICD-10-CM code set, additional coding concepts have been added.

U Codes

You will notice there are no U codes in ICD-10-CM. This was done on purpose. The World Health Organization has reserved all U codes for future use.

Placeholder Codes

ICD-9 allowed for placeholder codes, by using a zero. In an alphanumeric system, using zero could easily become confusing (as zero could be confused for O, and O for zero). Placeholder codes in ICD-10-CM are now signified with an X. You will most often see the placeholder codes in a section where anatomical reference or site is not used. The best example is in poisoning (T30-T50).

T49.2X1A Poisoning by local astringents and local detergents, accidental (unintentional), initial encounter

Combination Codes

Grouping conditions into one code is not a new coding concept. Combo codes exist in ICD-9. However, in ICD-10-CM, the idea is taken to a whole new level of intensity and specificity.

A combination code is simply one code used to denote two or more diagnoses, or a diagnosis with a specific manifestation, or a diagnosis with complications.

The most referenced examples of combination codes are the new Diabetes Mellitus codes (as mentioned before, typically found in the E08-E11 code ranges).

E10.21 – Type 1 Diabetes Mellitus with Diabetic Nephropathy

E10.341 – Type 1 diabetes mellitus with severe nonproliferative diabetic retinopathy with macular edema

E11.621 – Type 2 diabetes mellitus with foot ulcer

To identify when a combination code may be appropriate, look to the inclusion and exclusion notes which accompany the code set. Codes and other people engaged in the claims payment side of health care economics will need to work with clinical teams to closely identify where documentation can be improved to identify the possibility of combination codes. Insurance payers may deny claims that have multiple diagnosis codes attached that could, and likely should, have been combined together into one code.

Examples of documentation tips for common areas where combination codes are found could include:

Diabetes
Include type of diabetes, other systems that may be affected, and complications

Pressure Ulcers
Include stage, precise anatomical location, and number of ulcers

Injuries
Include the any loss of consciousness and specific cause of the injury

Examples:
- fall on same level
- motor vehicle accident
- animal bite (always document animal species)

Coders will need to partner with clinical teams to ensure all of the required information needed to document the proper code is present in the medical record. If the possibility of a combination code exists, the coder will need to query the physician for clarification. Clinicians who document well will assist the process, and reduce the cause of payment delays from CMS and other payers.

Excludes Notes

Excludes notes are not a new concept for ICD-10. A type of excludes notes existed in ICD-9. However, in ICD-10, there are two types of excludes notes.

Excludes notes can seem complicated to non-coders. However, they break down into fairly simple concepts.

Excludes Notes 1 – Type 1 Excludes Notes are the same as ICD-9 Excludes Notes. It means "not coded here." The Excludes Note indicates that a code is excluded and should not be included with the specific code you are reviewing. This is used to identify when two conditions cannot occur at once or together. A common example of this would be a congenital and an acquired version of the same condition.

Excludes Notes 2 – Type 2 Excludes Notes are used to mean "not included here." This means that the condition is not part of the condition under which it is listed. This is an important distinction because the second code, the one excluded from the first code, can be a separate and altogether different condition than the first. Both conditions can be present at once, but would need to be designated with both codes.

A common example of this would be a contusion to a specific body part (ankle). The excludes 2 on the ankle contusion may show contusion to the toes. So that means the ankle contusion does not include toe contusion. If the patient has both ankle and toe contusions, then both codes would need to be present.

BREAKDOWN OF ICD-10-CM CHAPTERS

- **A00-B99** Certain infectious and parasitic diseases
- **C00-D49** Neoplasms
- **D50-D89** Diseases of the blood and blood-forming organs and certain disorders involving the immune mechanism
- **E00-E89** Endocrine, nutritional and metabolic diseases
- **F01-F99** Mental, Behavioral and Neurodevelopmental disorders
- **G00-G99** Diseases of the nervous system
- **H00-H59** Diseases of the eye and adnexa
- **H60-H95** Diseases of the ear and mastoid process
- **I00-I99** Diseases of the circulatory system
- **J00-J99** Diseases of the respiratory system
- **K00-K95** Diseases of the digestive system
- **L00-L99** Diseases of the skin and subcutaneous tissue
- **M00-M99** Diseases of the musculoskeletal system and connective tissue
- **N00-N99** Diseases of the genitourinary system
- **O00-O9A** Pregnancy, childbirth and the puerperium
- **P00-P96** Certain conditions originating in the perinatal period
- **Q00-Q99** Congenital malformations, deformations and chromosomal abnormalities
- **R00-R99** Symptoms, signs and abnormal clinical and laboratory findings, not elsewhere classified
- **S00-T88** Injury, poisoning and certain other consequences of external causes
- **V00-Y99** External causes of morbidity
- **Z00-Z99** Factors influencing health status and contact with health services

Some of the largest Chapters (by volume of codes) are quite obvious. When you think about the added concepts listed earlier in the book, added considerations like laterality, instance, and healing of fractures, it is no surprise that the largest section of codes in the ICD-10-CM is Chapter 19.

Here are a few of the largest chapters in ICD-10-CM (by volume of codes):

Chapter	Code Range	Approximate # of Codes	Code Title
13	M00-M99	6,300+	Diseases of the musculoskeletal system and connective tissue (includes many uses of laterality)
15	O00-O9A	2,150+	Pregnancy, Childbirth, and the Puerperium (many codes include a trimester identifier)
19	S00-T88	39,860+	Injury, poisoning and certain other consequences of external causes (an obvious Chapter that uses etiology, laterality, open vs closed, union vs malunion, and detailed anatomical reference)

ICD-10-PCS

In the United States, a group of ICD-10 related procedure codes were developed. This code set is known as the ICD-10-PCS, or Procedural Coding System.

The PCS is not used for outpatient or physician settings. It is a group of procedure codes used by hospitals for inpatient reporting of procedures.

You may not be aware, but the ICD-9 code set had a small set of procedure codes. Due to the code structure, ICD-10-PCS does not easily lend itself to a quick chart of categories or sections. The codes are broken down by digit – where each digit represents a component of the procedure that was completed.

ICD-10-PCS can be broken down into what are called "root operations." There are 31 root operations. These operations are terms that are generalized, as they are the first part of the code. As the code moves through its additional digits, more and more specificity to the procedure is gained.

The ICD-10-PCS was created in coordination between 3M and CMS. This code set is not widely used outside of the United States. The original code set was released for use in 1998. Since the ICD-9-CM included procedural codes, but the ICD-10-CM does not, the ICD-10-PCS code set has been selected as the code set for inpatient setting procedure codes.

ICD-10-PCS STRUCTURE

The ICD-10-PCS is a completely new methodology.

The immediate differences include:

ICD-9	ICD-10
3-4 numbers per code	7 alphanumeric characters per code
Codes are a fixed set in list form	Codes are built from components using tables
Generic anatomy	Detailed and specific anatomy
Approximately 4,000 codes	Approximately 72,000 codes

The structure to ICD-10 is a very logical progression from left-to-right. This is true for ICD-10-CM and ICD-10-PCS.

An ICD-10-PCS code is built from a series of tables with relevant components based on the Character Position (meaning 1 through 7). The available codes in subsequent tables change based on characters chosen. Coding the ICD-10-PCS is a lot like "picking your own adventure" through the tables of available components.

Some key features or characteristics of the code set include:
- Standardized clinical terminology
- Standardized level of specificity
- No diagnostic information
- No "not otherwise specified" (NOS) code options
- Characters can be made up of the numbers 0–9 and the alphabet (except I and O, because they are easily confused with the numbers 1 and 0)

STANDARDIZED CLINICAL TERMINOLOGY

Some words used by clinicians and health care professionals can have multiple meanings. This can cause confusion on what procedure was performed, or in the case of some words, which part of a procedure was performed.

The most quoted example of this comes from the CMS Guide to ICD-10-PCS. The word "excision" is given as an example. This word is currently used to describe many types of procedures. In ICD-10-PCS, the word only describes a "single, precise surgical objective defined as Cutting out or off, without replacement, a portion of a body part."

Another example is the term "debridement." This procedure is a process, by which a clinician moves through several steps. Those steps could include excision, extraction, irrigation, and extirpation.

ICD-10-PCS CHARACTER BREAKDOWN

Character	Character Title	Description of Character
1	Section	This is an overall placement of the type of procedure. Examples of the available options include: • Medical and Surgical • Obstetrics • Osteopathic • Chiropractic • Radiation Therapy • Mental Health • …and several more
2	Body System	This is the specific body system that is being impacted. When you select the first character, specific options are made available to you based on the Section you have selected. For example, Obstetrics has only one option (pregnancy), while Medical and Surgical has over 30 options (including central nervous system, upper arteries, eye, endocrine system, upper bones, male reproductive system, and several more).
3	Root Operation	The Root Operation is the "meat and potatoes" of the ICD-10-PCS code. This Character is the most talked about in available ICD-10 resources, as it drives what was specifically done to the patient. As mentioned above, there are 31 Root Operations. A list of these Root Operations has been provided in the next section of this book.

Character	Character Title	Description of Character
4	Body Part	This is the specific body part that is being impacted by the Root Operation.
5	Approach	Approach, like Body System, changes based on which Root Operation and Section are selected. Examples of Approach include: • Open • Percutaneous Endoscopic; • Via Natural or Artificial Opening Endoscopic • Endoscopic Assistance • External • Radionuclide • Contrast (high/low osmolar contrast) • …and several more
6	Device	When appropriate for the procedure, the Device Character is used to indicate which device was used. Examples can include Isotope (for Radiation) or Substance (for Administration). As with other Characters, the Device character is dependent on other selections in the overall code.
7	Qualifier	This Character is used much like the ICD-10-CM 7th Character Extension. As with other Characters, the Qualifier character is dependent on other selections in the overall code. An example of the Qualifier character can be found in indicating if a biopsy was diagnostic or therapeutic. An "X" is selected if the reason for the procedure is diagnostic, and a "Z" is selected if the procedure is therapeutic.

LIST OF ICD-10-PCS ROOT OPERATIONS

Below you will find a list of the 31 Root Operations that drive the methodology in appropriately coding for ICD-10-PCS.

Alteration	Division	Inspection	Reposition
Bypass	Drainage	Map	Resection
Change	Excision	Occlusion	Restriction
Control	Extirpation	Reattachment	Revision
Creation	Extraction	Release	Supplement
Destruction	Fragmentation	Removal	Transfer
Detachment	Fusion	Repair	Transplantation
Dilation	Insertion	Replacement	

COMMON MYTHS DE-MYTH-STIFIED

Since the announcement that the HHS was requiring the United States health care system to move onto ICD-10, there has been a lot of speculation and commentary. Many websites have cropped up that generate traffic and panic by claiming that the most outlandish requirements are going to be levied onto physicians and other clinicians. Groups, such as the American Medical Association (AMA), have released many statements about the negative impact ICD-10 could have on physicians and other providers.

At the end of the day, ICD-10 is an inevitability. The United States is already cross-mapping reported ICD-9 codes into ICD-10 codes and reporting those to the international medical community. Many software companies have accommodated ICD-10 in updates and rollouts, so that impacts to electronic medical records and claims processing platforms would be minimal.

Change is tough.

Below you will read about some myths that have been spread about ICD-10, and then you will read the truth of the situation.

Myth 1: We will get another extension
A common belief is that the Department of Health and Human Services will delay the implementation of ICD-10 again. There is also a belief that the American Medical Association, and assorted other special interest groups with lobbying powers in Washington D.C., will convince the United States Congress to push the implementation out again.

Truth: That is not happening. ICD-10 is set to implement on October 1st, 2015.

Myth 2: Too many codes!
The first attach on ICD-10 to crop up is that the additional level of required specificity in the code set means that no one will be able to use the system – there are simply too many codes.

Truth: The best answer to this came directly from CMS.

"Just as an increase in the number of words in a dictionary doesn't make it more difficult to use, the greater number of codes in ICD-10-CM/PCS doesn't necessarily make it more complex to use. In fact, the greater number of codes in ICD-10-CM/PCS make it easier for you to find the right code. In addition, just as you don't have to search the entire list of ICD-9-CM codes for the proper code, you also don't have to conduct searches of the entire list of ICD-10-CM/PCS codes. The Alphabetic Index and electronic coding tools are available to help you select the proper code. The improved structure and specificity of ICD-10-CM/PCS will likely assist in developing increasingly sophisticated electronic coding tools that will help you more quickly select codes. Because ICD-10-CM/PCS is much more specific, is more clinically accurate, and uses a more logical structure, it is much easier to use than ICD-9-CM. Most physician practices use a relatively small number of diagnosis codes that are generally related to a specific type of specialty."

This is likely CMS' version of a mic drop.

Myth 3: TOO Specific!

ICD-10 will require way too much documentation. The medical records will be way too detailed. This is an unnecessary administrative burden on clinicians.

Truth: The information necessary to properly code in ICD-10 is clinical information that physicians and other health care providers should already be documenting in the medical record.

Earlier in the book you read about increased specificity, with the example of a broken arm. A physician who refuses to document which arm is broken, or a radiology tech who does not notate on the scan which arm was scanned, is a poor clinician indeed. The specificity requirements in ICD-10 are reasonable, as they apply directly to patient care.

Yes, some of the codes can become obnoxious, like T71.231 (Asphyxiation due to being trapped in a discarded refrigerator, accidental), or W49.01 (Hair causing external constriction), but remember that the original purpose of the ICD was to record statistics surrounding death. The code set is still used for that purpose by many countries.

CMS has released guidance that injury and historical codes (like the two examples shown above) will continue to follow the same requirements that were in place for ICD-9.

What most of the naysayers aren't saying is that ICD-9 had these types of codes too (994.7 Asphyxiation by bunny bag. E928.4 external constriction caused by hair)!

Myth 4: ICD-10 will cause waste and abuse!
There is an assumption that greater specificity in coding means that health care professionals are going to be required to increase the diagnostic testing done to move from a differential diagnosis to a specific diagnosis.

Truth: The guidance from CMS is quite clear this is not a concern.

"As with ICD-9-CM, ICD-10-CM codes are derived from documentation in the medical record. Therefore, if a diagnosis has not yet been established, you should code the condition to its highest degree of certainty (which may be a sign or symptom) when using both coding systems. In fact, ICD-10-CM contains many more codes for signs and symptoms than ICD-9-CM, and it is better designed for use in ambulatory encounters when definitive diagnoses are often not yet known. Nonspecific codes are still available in ICD-10-CM/PCS for use when more detailed clinical information is not known."

Myth 5: CPT codes are changing!
Truth: ICD-10 will not change the CPT or HCPCS code set (as discussed earlier in the book). ICD-10-PCS is only used for inpatient facility coding of procedures that are done in an inpatient setting.

IMPLEMENTATION DATE AND IMPORTANT POINTS

Depending on when you are reading this book, the ICD-10 implementation date may have come and gone, or you may be cramming before the big day. The current implementation date for ICD-10 in the United States is October 1st, 2015.

Knowing the transition date is important because that will define how you read medical claims based on which code is required.

ICD-9	Any claim that has a date of service, or date of discharge, before October 1st, 2015, will be coded in ICD-9.
ICD-10	ICD-10 Any claim that has a date of service, or date of discharge, on or after October 1st, 2015, will be coded in ICD-10.

Most payers, and the guidance from CMS, state that claims which will straddle the two dates should be broken into two claims; one for ICD-9, and one for ICD-10.

As you can imagine, there are a lot of "what-if" scenarios that could come up in dealing with such a hard and fast rule. CMS has release a series of articles, based on specialty, for how to handle what it calls "claims that span the ICD-10 implementation date." These resource can help you work through the "what-if" scenarios you may run into.

THE GREATEST IMPACT OF ICD-10

ICD-10 implementation will cause a lot of ripples through the entire health care community. Impacts will include Insurance Companies/Payers rejecting claims based on their interpretation of the ICD-10 guidelines, Physicians and other clinicians being queried over and over on the same patient's condition, and plenty of other administrative areas.

However, arguably the biggest impact to be caused by ICD-10 is in clinical documentation. The way physicians, nurses, dieticians, respiratory therapists, and countless other clinicians document a patient's heal in the medical record is the crux of how ICD-10 operates.

Convincing physicians and other clinicians to include a great level of detail in their documented findings will be the true hurdle for most business offices, billing departments, or health information management teams.

This area has been a major focus of various special interest groups and other agencies (like the AMA) in stating that the administrative burden placed on physicians will be great. People on the other side of the argument focus on the ability to improve patient care through the level of detail required in ICD-10.

ICD-10 is not meant as a way to force providers to change their Clinical Documentation will see the greatest impact during transition to ICD-10. Coders will need a deeper understanding of anatomy and physiology, and physicians and other clinicians will be required to ensure all relevant information is fully documented.

After all, the Golden Rule of patient care is: "If it wasn't documented, it wasn't done."

The two major things to keep in mind about the new clinical documentation requirements in ICD-10:

- ICD-10 is not changing clinical assessment skills. Instead, the code set will require more fully documented proof of the normal problems, assessments, procedures, and treatments.

- The provider query process for inpatient stays is a pre-discharge requirement. Clinicians can no longer add to a medical record after a patient has been discharged and expect to be paid for those medical claims. Documentation needs to occur as the patient is being treated.

In 2011, CMS released a bulletin with a list of areas where documentation specificity requirements may be more challenging. The list included a series of "diagnosis types" and associated areas of required documentation. Some of those areas are covered below, with additional information and tips that have come out since 2011.

Many groups of physician specialties have released statements on how to properly document and code for common diagnosis (in those specialties). Those resources are available for physicians who are focused in one area of medicine (Chiropractic, Behavioral Health, Nephrology, and others).

AREAS OF CHALLENGE IN CLINICAL DOCUMENTATION

The following list will give you a general idea of what to expect when looking to improve clinical documentation. Like you can find within the code set, there are a lot of repetitive considerations below. Once you have a handle on these basics, you should be well on your way to affect some positive change in the clinical documentation you encounter.

Diabetes Mellitus

ICD-9 has a total of 59 codes for diabetes. ICD-10 has more than 200 codes. These additional codes include additional types of diabetes, complications, and encounter information. There are also many choices for potential combination codes within the E08-E11 code set. Understanding when a comorbidity moves from being listed as a separate diagnosis, and when it is directly tied to another diagnosis, will be a challenge all on its own.

Here are a few areas of focused documentation for Diabetes Mellitus:
- Include the Type of Diabetes (underlying, gestational, etc)
- Identify all Body systems affected (oral, skin, joint, etc)
- Is the diagnosis a complication or manifestation (skin ulcer, neuropathy)
- Signify the Patient Encounter (initial, subsequent, sequela)

ICD-10 codes are expanded to include the classification and then manifestation in one code. The coding category has been updated with current clinical classifications, and does not rely on "Juvenile and Adult-Onset" terms (which are outdated and not clinically accurate). Also, simply documenting "controlled" versus "uncontrolled" is not enough information to properly code the diagnosis in ICD-10.

Injuries

ICD-10 features an expanded category for injuries. The seventh character extension identifies a range of additional information, including the encounter type. Examples of this seventh character extension in the coding of injuries could include:

- "A" for the initial encounter
- "D" for the subsequent encounter for fracture with routine healing
- "G" for subsequent encounter for fracture with delayed healing
- "S" for sequela

Here are a few areas of focused documentation for injuries:
- Size and depth of the injury (example: lacerations)
- Anatomical Site – bone, muscle, joint, nerve involved
- Laterality
- Patient Encounter
- The specific Cause of the injury

A note about Cause

There has been a lot of debate about the use of "cause" in clinical documentation and coding in ICD-10. This is where much of the commentary surrounding "crazy" codes has generated. However, most of the "cause" codes are used for additional information purposes, and as you read earlier in this book, those codes existed even in ICD-9.

Documenting cause is a part of ensuring proper patient care. The idea that a broken arm from a sports injury, and a broken arm due to osteoporosis would be treated the same is not clinically sound. These factors are taken into consideration by a clinician during treatment, and thus should be documented as part of the diagnosis and treatment planning.

Documenting Cause could easily include the follow types of detail:
- How, where, and when the accident or injury occurred
- Loss of consciousness at the time of the injury
- Level of consciousness when presented for treatment
- Anatomic site of the injury, including laterality
- Type of injury
- Severity of injury

Each of those factors would be taken into consideration when treating an injury. It is easy to get caught up in the "now ICD-10 has codes for accidents in Outer Space.

Fractures

Fractures are a type of injury, however there are additional levels of documentation required for fractures that you will not see in other injury types.

Here are a few areas of focused documentation for fractures:
- Precise nature of the fracture type
  (joint involvement, fracture pattern, pathological or traumatic)
- Specific anatomical site, including laterality
- Fracture classification (open or closed)
  - Closed: Salter Harris Classification System
  - Open: Gustilo Classification System
- Displaced or nondisplaced
- Healing on subsequent encounters
  (normal, delayed, nonunion, malunion)

Drug Under-dosing

Under-dosing is a new concept for medical diagnostic coding. This code is used when a patient is non-compliant to medication, dietary, and other prescribed therapies. The under-dosing diagnosis code is not a primary diagnosis (it is always listed as secondary). This code is used to explain why the patient is not taking the medication or following the therapy.

Here are a few areas of focused documentation for under-dosing:
- List whether the under-dosing was intentional or unintentional
- Reason for the under-dosing (this can be things like financial hardship, related to a condition or other diagnosis, age-related debility, etc.)

Pregnancy

Here are a few areas of focused documentation for pregnancy:
- Trimester
  (pregnancy codes often require the trimester at the time of encounter)
  - First trimester, less than 14 weeks 0 days
  - Second trimester, 14 weeks 0 days through less than 28 weeks 0 days
  - Third trimester, 28 weeks 0 days until delivery
- Identifier if first pregnancy
- Pre-existing conditions
- Number of fetus (up to a fifth fetus)
  (this is a new component to coding in ICD-10)

Diagnosis Documentation Considerations

As you have reviewed the various chapters in this book, a few underlying themes should be obvious. ICD-10 is about greater specificity in coding, which drives better clinical documentation, to prove that quality patient care was achieved.

When interacting with the ICD-10 code set, there are a few key considerations to keep in mind. These topics will help you in properly coding, documenting, or understanding the codes and coding systems.

Remember:
- Any functional impairment or complications experienced
- Phase or stage of illness or injury
- Lateralization and detailed anatomical location
- Instance or episode of care (primary or subsequent)
- Any known co-morbidities
- Manifestations
- Etiology (cause)
- Sequela (in relation to another diagnosis)

MAKING IT MANAGEABLE

Now that you know more about ICD-10, how do you wrap your head around how to implement it into your work?

Here are a few thoughts to keep in mind:

- While there are thousands of new codes in ICD-10, there are not thousands of new diseases.

   Patterns exist in the code set that makes it seem larger.

   Over 1/3 of the codes are repeated codes where laterality is the only difference

   The codes are a repeating system that are similar from code to code with variations on one or two concepts (encounter, laterality, routine or delayed healing, malunion, nonunion, etc.)

- Do not allow yourself to become overcome with the vast number of codes. Start with a focus on your clinical domain.

   Each clinician has a specialty, and even those who are generalists see certain conditions or diseases regularly. Start by becoming familiar with the coding and documentation requirements for those conditions or diseases. Then branch out to additional codes that represent diagnoses you come across, just left frequently.

RESOURCES

As mentioned earlier in this book, there are a lot of available resources. The links below are reputable sources for information on ICD-10-CM and ICD-10-PCS.

https://www.cms.gov/Medicare/Coding/ICD10/index.html is a great website with a variety of tools and resources available for a wide range of provider, payer, and health care professionals. CMS also offers some useful interactive case studies that can be used to help team members calibrate on what the expectation is in ICD-10, and how far your team needs to go to get there.

http://www.icd10data.com is a free online resource that breaks down the code set into manageable chunks. The site is well annotated, and shows inclusions, exclusions 1 and 2, and other useful points of information for coding accurately in ICD-10 (like synonyms of disease names). In addition, when you become familiar with navigating the website, you will notice that some mapping of old ICD-9 codes into ICD-10 codes can be found. This should not be used to replace traditional and formal forward mapping, but it is a good resource to help "check your work" when you are moving from one code set to another.

For Providers – beyond the tools available on the CMS website, you should work closely with your payers. Understanding what your payers are looking for can greatly reduce the cost of claims resubmissions and delayed payments.

For Coders – AAPC and AHIMA have extensive training available to help you reach certification or familiar with ICD-10. There are also a variety of Facebook and LinkedIn groups that bring together coders from various backgrounds to help one another with complicated (or not so complicated) coding questions.

WRAP-UP

ICD-10 has been delayed for so long in the United States that it has generated a storm of publicity which has detracted from the truth of the code set. ICD-10 is not a new CMS creation that is sent to over-complicate the health care system. It is a standardized set of diagnosis codes (along with a new and improved inpatient procedural coding system) meant to streamline reporting and eliminate questions caused by an outdated system.

The implementation of ICD-10 is not as scary as you have heard. The implementation will require work. There will be a definite learning curve as the United States moves away from a code set it has used since the cancellation of "Gunsmoke" the television program in the 1970s. And if you are reading this after the October 1st, 2015 implementation date, then you can assure yourself that the world did not end because of ICD-10.

Patient care is the purpose of medicine. The United States moved away from documenting patient care in its use of ICD-9. Now, with ICD-10, you have a chance to implement rules and processes that will ensure quality patient care is documented and reimbursed in claims payment.

So while there are tens of thousands of new codes, you now know that the system relies on repeating concepts like laterality, anatomical location, and combination codes of two or more diseases. The tens of thousands of new codes are manageable. The processes of taking a differential diagnosis and working to a specific diagnosis has not changed. There are not additional testing requirements just to rule out all possibilities.

Clinical assessment skills do not need to change. Physicians and other clinicians need to do a better job at recording pertinent facts. Medical billers and coders need to do a better job at finding specific codes instead of using unspecified for everything.

Good luck in implementing ICD-10 for your office, team, department, or company. You are not alone, and there is help out there. Use the information you learned in this book to help you navigate the system of blogs, websites, books, and other content.

After all, if nations without access to Google.com and the Internet in general can implement ICD-10, then one of the most technologically advanced nations in the World can get through implementation with only minimal impact.